COMPLETE GUIDE TO UNDERSTANDING APPENDECTOMY

Essential Insights, Procedures, Recovery Tips, And Patient Care For Optimal Health Outcomes

KLEIN HOYLE

© [KLEIN HOYLE] [2024]

All rights reserved.

No part of this book may be reproduced, distributed, or transmitted in any form or by any means, including photocopying, recording, or other electronic or mechanical methods, without the publisher's prior written permission, with the exception of brief quotations in critical reviews and certain other noncommercial uses permitted by copyright law.

Disclaimer

The content in this book is based on the author's expertise and comprehension of the topic. The author has no affiliation or link with any corporation, business, or person. This book is meant to give general information and educational material only, and it should not be interpreted as professional medical advice. Always seek the advice of a skilled healthcare expert if you have any queries about medical issues or treatments. The author and publisher expressly disclaim any responsibility resulting directly or indirectly from the use or use of the information included in this book.

Table of Contents

ABOUT THIS BOOK

The "Complete Guide to Understanding Appendectomy" is an invaluable resource for medical professionals, patients, and anybody looking for in-depth information on this frequent surgical treatment. This book is a comprehensive compilation that covers every element of appendectomy, from its historical background to current methods, offering a clear awareness of its importance and procedures.

The first chapters expose readers to the foundations of appendectomy, including its definition, purpose, and historical history. Understanding the most frequent causes of having an appendectomy emphasizes the significance of prompt treatment, laying the groundwork for the crucial information that follows.

This book is built on an in-depth examination of the appendix's anatomy, which explains its structure, function, and susceptibility to different illnesses. This section provides readers with a good basis for understanding appendicitis symptoms, including early indicators, symptom development, and differential diagnosis, emphasizing the need for early identification.

The diagnosis process is rigorously thorough, including a medical history, physical examination, and a variety of laboratory and imaging procedures. This book explains the diagnostic procedure, allowing readers to understand the necessity of correct and fast diagnosis in appendicitis care.

Appendectomy preparation, including pre-operative instructions, surgical choices, and risk-benefit analysis, is extensively investigated to assuage patient anxieties and guarantee informed decision-making. Step-by-step instructions for the surgical process, anesthesia procedures, and post-operative care protocols give a thorough road map for both patients and healthcare personnel.

This book also goes into the complexities of post-operative care, leading readers through the early recovery period, pain management tactics, wound care regimens, and being alert for any problems. It also explains the long-term recovery pathway, which includes physiotherapy, nutritional concerns, and follow-up care to optimize results.

A separate chapter on complications and hazards emphasizes the significance of monitoring in post-operative care, enabling readers to identify, react to, and prevent any bad outcomes. Special considerations for vulnerable groups, such as children, pregnant women, and the elderly, are also made, assuring inclusion and targeted care delivery.

To summarise, the "Complete Guide to Understanding Appendectomy" is a thorough compendium that goes beyond its title, providing a holistic view of appendicitis treatment from diagnosis to long-term care. This book is a useful resource for healthcare professionals and patients alike, as it distills complicated medical ideas into understandable insights, allowing for informed decision-making and optimum results.

CHAPTER 1

Introduction To Appendectomy

Definition And Purpose Of Appendectomy

An appendectomy is a surgical surgery that removes the appendix, which is a tiny pouch connected to the large intestine. The goal of this procedure is to treat appendicitis, which is an inflammation of the appendix. The appendix serves no fundamental role in the body, hence removing it has no negative consequences or substantial alterations in basic processes.

The appendix may become inflamed for a variety of causes, including fecal obstruction, infection, and tumors. When the appendix gets inflamed, it causes severe stomach pain, nausea, vomiting, and fever. If left untreated, it might burst, resulting in potentially fatal consequences such as peritonitis, an inflammation of the abdominal lining.

Appendectomy is the main therapy for appendicitis, and it is often done as soon as the illness is detected. The procedure seeks to remove the inflamed appendix before it ruptures, eliminating future problems and allowing the patient to recuperate more quickly.

A Brief History Of Appendectomy

Appendectomy has a long history, dating back to 1886 when pathologist Dr. Reginald Fitz characterized the ailment of appendicitis for the first time. He recognized appendix inflammation as a unique medical disease requiring surgical intervention.

Dr. William W. Grant performed the first successful appendectomy in Iowa, USA, in 1889. The procedure gained widespread acceptance and popularity after Dr. Charles McBurney, an American surgeon, published a landmark paper in 1889 outlining a specific technique for removing the appendix, now known as the McBurney incision.

Since then, appendectomy has become one of the most popular surgical operations done across the globe, with advances in surgical methods and technology resulting in safer and more successful patient outcomes.

Common Reasons For Appendectomy

The most frequent cause of an appendectomy is appendicitis, which is when the appendix becomes inflamed. This inflammation may be induced by many sources, including:

• Blockage from feces, foreign objects, or parasites may cause inflammation and infection in the appendix.

• Bacterial infections may induce inflammation in the appendix, resulting in appendicitis.

• Tumours in the appendix may induce blockage and inflammation, resulting in appendicitis.

Appendicitis symptoms often include acute stomach discomfort, particularly in the lower right quadrant, nausea, vomiting, and fever. Prompt diagnosis and treatment are critical to avoiding complications including rupture and peritonitis.

Importance Of Timely Intervention

Early management in instances of appendicitis is critical for avoiding major complications and promoting a quick recovery. If left untreated, appendicitis may rupture the appendix, allowing infectious debris to enter the abdominal cavity and cause peritonitis, a potentially fatal illness.

The most effective therapy for appendicitis is surgical removal of the inflamed appendix (appendectomy). By removing the appendix before it ruptures, doctors may minimize infection spread and lower the risk of consequences.

Prompt diagnosis and surgical intervention also reduce hospitalization and recuperation time for patients, enabling them to return to routine activities sooner. Furthermore, early treatment lowers the risk of complications and provides a better prognosis for the patient. As a result, recognizing appendicitis symptoms and receiving medical assistance as soon as possible is critical to a positive outcome.

CHAPTER 2

Anatomy Of The Appendix

Location And Structure Of The Appendix

The appendix is a tiny, finger-shaped pouch found at the intersection of the small and large intestines. It is commonly found in the lower right abdomen, however the specific location varies significantly between people. The appendix is a short, tubular organ with a closed-end, similar to a little worm or finger.

Despite its small size, the appendix plays an important function in the immune system. Its structure contains lymphatic tissue, which aids in the generation of antibodies and white blood cells, aiding the body's defense against illnesses.

Understanding the location and anatomy of the appendix is critical for identifying and treating appendicitis, which is a frequent illness of this organ. Its closeness to other abdominal organs, as well as its distinctive anatomy, might impact the symptoms of appendicitis.

The Function Of The Appendix

While the specific function of the human appendix is still contested, it is thought to have a role in the immune system. The lymphatic tissue in the appendix aids in the development of antibodies and white blood cells, which are critical components of the body's defense against illnesses.

Some researchers also believe that the appendix may operate as a reservoir for beneficial bacteria, assisting in the regeneration of gut flora after infections that deplete the intestinal microbiota. However, the loss of the appendix does not seem to have a major negative impact on general health, showing that although its function may be advantageous, it is not required for life.

Understanding the appendix's function sheds light on its relevance in general health and its possible role in particular medical diseases, such as appendicitis.

Common Disorders Of The Appendix

Appendicitis is the most frequent appendix condition. It happens when the appendix becomes inflamed, which is usually caused by fecal waste, foreign substances, or, in rare circumstances, tumors obstructing its lumen. Appendicitis symptoms often include stomach discomfort, nausea, vomiting, and fever.

If left untreated, appendicitis may cause complications such as appendix perforation, which can lead to peritonitis, a severe infection of the abdominal cavity. Prompt diagnosis and treatment, often in the form of surgical removal of the appendix (appendectomy), are critical to avoiding complications and ensuring a positive result.

Appendiceal tumors, such as carcinoid tumors or adenocarcinomas, are less prevalent illnesses that affect the appendix and may need surgical excision.

Understanding the most prevalent appendix illnesses is critical for recognizing symptoms and obtaining medical assistance promptly to avoid complications and allow proper treatment.

Diagnostic Procedures For Appendix Issues

Several diagnostic procedures are used to evaluate appendix problems, including appendicitis. This includes:

1. **Physical Examination:** A healthcare professional may do a physical examination to examine the patient's symptoms, with a focus on abdominal soreness, rebound tenderness, and the presence of guarding or stiffness, all of which indicate abdominal inflammation.

2. Blood tests, such as a complete blood count (CBC) and inflammatory markers like C-reactive protein (CRP) and white blood cell count (WBC), may be used to detect symptoms of infection and inflammation.

3. Imaging Studies: Ultrasound or computed tomography (CT) scans may be performed to see the appendix and look for symptoms of inflammation or blockage. These imaging investigations may assist in confirming the diagnosis of appendicitis and guide surgical treatment.

4. Diagnostic Laparoscopy: When the diagnosis is unknown, diagnostic laparoscopy—a minimally invasive surgical procedure—may be used to directly see the appendix and check for inflammation or other abnormalities. This method enables both diagnosis and treatment, since an appendectomy may be done if appendicitis is proven.

Understanding the diagnostic tools for appendix disorders is critical for healthcare personnel to effectively detect and treat illnesses such as appendicitis, allowing for prompt intervention and better patient outcomes.

CHAPTER 3

Symptoms Of Appendicitis

Early Signs Of Appendicitis

Recognizing the early indications of appendicitis is critical for receiving timely medical care and treatment. The most frequent early symptom is abdominal discomfort, which often begins at the belly button and progresses to the lower right side of the abdomen. This discomfort ranges from mild to acute and may intensify with movement, coughing, or sneezing. Individuals may also feel a lack of appetite, nausea, vomiting, and a mild temperature.

It is crucial to remember that the early symptoms of appendicitis may be mild and readily misdiagnosed as other illnesses. Some folks may dismiss their pain as indigestion or a temporary stomach virus. However, if you have chronic abdomen discomfort or any of these symptoms, get medical attention right once.

Symptom Progression

As appendicitis advances, the symptoms usually become more acute and apparent. The abdominal discomfort worsens and becomes focused in the lower right quadrant of the abdomen. The discomfort may become chronic and severe, making it difficult to move or walk comfortably.

In addition to increased pain, additional symptoms may emerge, including:

• Appendicitis may cause a low-grade fever due to the body's inflammatory reaction.

• Changes in bowel habits: Individuals may have constipation, diarrhea, or both.

• Increased stomach soreness, particularly in the lower right quadrant.

As the infection develops, the appendix may swell and fill with pus, resulting in an appendiceal abscess. In extreme situations, the appendix may burst, resulting in peritonitis, a potentially fatal abdominal infection.

Differential Diagnosis

Several other illnesses may produce symptoms identical to appendicitis, making diagnosis difficult. Differential diagnosis is critical for ruling out other possible causes of stomach discomfort. Some conditions that might resemble appendicitis are:

- **Gastroenteritis:** Inflammation of the stomach and intestines caused by viral or bacterial infection may result in abdominal discomfort, nausea, vomiting, and diarrhea.

- Urinary tract infections (UTIs) in the bladder or kidneys may cause lower abdomen discomfort and symptoms include urgency, frequency, and burning feeling while urinating.

- Women may have stomach discomfort owing to ovarian cysts or torsion.

- IBD, such as Crohn's disease or ulcerative colitis, may cause persistent inflammation of the gastrointestinal system, resulting in stomach discomfort, diarrhea, and other symptoms.

The Importance Of Early Detection

Early identification of appendicitis is crucial for avoiding complications and receiving prompt treatment. Delayed diagnosis or treatment may cause the appendix to burst, resulting in peritonitis, a serious and possibly fatal infection of the abdomen. Prompt detection of symptoms and medical examination are critical for avoiding problems and facilitating a speedier recovery.

Furthermore, misinterpretation of appendicitis might result in needless medications or surgical procedures for illnesses that have similar symptoms. As a result, healthcare personnel use a mix of clinical examination, laboratory testing, and imaging investigations to properly diagnose and distinguish appendicitis from other comparable illnesses.

In conclusion, recognizing the early indicators of appendicitis, understanding the course of symptoms, evaluating differential diagnoses, and emphasizing the need for early discovery are all critical parts of properly treating this illness. Being aware of these characteristics allows people to seek immediate medical care and get appropriate treatment, lowering the risk of problems and facilitating a speedier recovery.

CHAPTER 4

Diagnosis Of Appendicitis

Medical History And Physical Examination

A comprehensive medical history and a careful physical examination are often used to diagnose appendicitis. Your doctor will ask you about your symptoms, such as when they began, how severe they are, and where you are experiencing discomfort. They will also ask about your medical history, particularly any past abdominal procedures or diseases that may resemble appendicitis.

During the physical exam, your doctor will gently palpate your abdomen to detect pain and inflammation. They may also conduct tests such as the rebound tenderness test, which involves applying pressure to the abdomen and then releasing it to determine whether the pain increases—a typical symptom of appendicitis. They may also examine for other symptoms such as fever, nausea, and vomiting, which are frequent in appendicitis patients.

Lab Tests

Laboratory testing is essential for verifying an appendicitis diagnosis. Blood tests, such as a complete blood count (CBC), might show high white blood cell counts, indicating an infection or inflammation in the body. Elevated levels of specific indicators, such as CRP and lactate, may help confirm the diagnosis of appendicitis.

Urine tests may also be performed to rule out other illnesses that produce similar symptoms, such as a urinary tract infection. These tests serve to narrow down the options and give useful information to aid in diagnosis.

Imaging Techniques

In certain situations, further imaging examinations are required to establish the diagnosis of appendicitis and rule out alternative possibilities. Ultrasound, CT scans, and MRI are popular imaging procedures in this setting.

Ultrasound utilizes sound waves to produce pictures of the abdominal region, enabling clinicians to see the appendix and look for symptoms of inflammation, such as thickening of the wall or fluid surrounding it. It is a non-invasive and rapid technique that may give vital information about the illness.

CT scans are more comprehensive imaging investigations that show cross-sections of the abdomen. They provide a thorough image of the appendix and surrounding tissues, allowing clinicians to detect any anomalies or problems related to appendicitis.

MRI, albeit less frequent than ultrasonography and CT scans, may be used to visualize the appendix and detect inflammation. It is especially effective in situations when radiation exposure must be minimized, such as in pregnant women or children.

Confirming The Diagnosis

Once the medical history, physical examination, and diagnostic testing are finished, the healthcare team will carefully review the results to confirm the diagnosis of appendicitis. A mix of clinical judgment and test data is usually utilized to achieve an accurate diagnosis.

If appendicitis is diagnosed, immediate treatment is required to avoid complications including perforation or abscess development. In rare circumstances, particularly when the diagnosis is unknown, hospitalization may be indicated to monitor symptoms and determine if surgery is necessary.

Overall, diagnosing appendicitis requires a thorough approach that includes a medical history, physical examination, laboratory testing, and imaging modalities to achieve a clear conclusion and begin appropriate therapy. Early detection and care are critical to achieving positive outcomes for individuals with appendicitis.

CHAPTER 5

Preparing For Appendectomy

Preoperative Instructions For Patients

Medical Examination and Testing

Before having an appendectomy, patients must have a full medical examination. This involves a thorough medical history review, a physical examination, and a variety of tests such as blood work, urine, and imaging procedures like an ultrasound or CT scan. These methods assist in confirming the diagnosis of appendicitis and rule out alternative possibilities.

Medication Adjustments

Patients should notify their healthcare practitioner about any medicines they are presently taking, including over-the-counter pharmaceuticals and vitamins.

Some medicines, notably blood thinners and anti-inflammatory drugs, may need to be stopped a few days before surgery to lessen the possibility of significant bleeding during the treatment.

Fasting and Dietary Restrictions

Patients are usually told not to eat or drink after midnight the night before their procedure. This fasting helps to avoid difficulties during anesthesia, such as aspiration, which occurs when stomach contents are inhaled into the lungs. The surgical team will offer specific dietary and hydration consumption advice.

Hygiene and Skin Preparations

Patients are often recommended to wash with antibacterial soap in the morning before surgery to lessen the chance of infection. They should also refrain from shaving the surgery region themselves to minimize skin irritation or infection; this will be done in a sterile setting if required.

Clothing & Personal Items

Patients should dress comfortably and loosely during their hospital visit. They should also leave valuables like jewelry, watches, and wallets at home. Bring identification, insurance information, and a list of current medicines to the hospital.

Transportation arrangements

Patients will be unable to drive themselves home following the operation due to the effects of anesthesia; thus, plans should be made for a responsible adult to transport them home and remain with them for the first 24 hours after surgery.

Appendectomy (Open vs. Laparoscopic)

Open appendectomy

An open appendectomy removes the appendix with a single, bigger incision in the lower right abdomen. This conventional method is often used when the appendix ruptures or there is extensive infection.

Procedure

1. An incision of 2-4 inches is created in the lower right abdomen.

2. Appendix Removal: The surgeon locates and delicately removes the appendix.

3. Closure: The incision is stitched or stapled.

Laparoscopic Appendectomy

A laparoscopic appendectomy is a minimally invasive operation that involves numerous tiny incisions and specialized devices, including a laparoscope, which is a thin tube equipped with a camera.

Procedure

1. Incisions: Several tiny incisions (typically three) are made in the stomach.

2. The laparoscope and other surgical equipment are introduced via these incisions.

3. Visualisation and Removal: The camera magnifies the appendix, which is subsequently removed using the equipment.

4. Closure: Small wounds are closed with stitches or surgical glue.

Comparative Overview

• Laparoscopic surgery often results in speedier recovery and less postoperative discomfort compared to open surgery.

• Minimal scarring from laparoscopic surgery owing to smaller incisions.

• Both procedures have low complication rates, although laparoscopic surgery tends to have less postoperative issues.

Risks And Benefits Of Surgery

Benefits

• Relief from Symptoms: Removing the inflamed appendix relieves severe abdominal discomfort caused by appendicitis.

• Appendectomy avoids appendix rupture, which may cause dangerous illnesses such as peritonitis and abscess development.

• Quick recovery: Laparoscopic surgery allows patients to resume regular activities within a week or two.

Risks

• Surgical procedures carry the risk of infection at incision sites and inside the abdomen.

• There is a risk of bleeding during or after surgery, although it is usually low.

• Rare but possible complications of anesthesia include breathing problems and allergic reactions.

• Surrounding organs may be injured during surgery.

Risk Management

To reduce these risks, surgeons adhere to stringent sterilization measures, use precise surgical methods, and constantly monitor patients during and after the treatment. Pre-operative assessments and attention to pre-surgery instructions are also important in lowering the risk of problems.

Consent And Psychological Preparation

Informed Consent

Before surgery, patients must offer informed consent. During this process, the surgeon explains the surgery, its aim, the risks and advantages, and any alternatives. Patients are encouraged to ask questions and clarify any confusion they may have.

The patient then signs the permission document, indicating that they understand and agree to the surgery.

Psychological Preparation

Preparing psychologically and emotionally for surgery is as vital as physical preparation. Patients should:

• Educate themselves: Knowing what to anticipate before and after surgery helps reduce anxiety. Reading informed materials or speaking with the surgical team might be beneficial.

• Openly discussing anxieties and concerns with healthcare professionals might bring comfort.

• Support System: Seeking emotional support from family and friends helps reduce stress. Knowing that loved ones are accessible might provide comfort.

• Deep breathing, meditation, and yoga may help lower anxiety before surgery.

Post-operative Planning

Patients should prepare for their recovery time by ensuring that they have a comfortable place to relax, required supplies such as medicines and bandages, and access to follow-up care. Preparing for assistance with everyday chores might also aid in a smooth recovery process.

Patients who prepare adequately, both physically and emotionally, may approach an appendectomy with confidence, lowering the risk of complications and facilitating a speedy recovery.

CHAPTER 6

The Appendectomy Procedure

Step-By-Step Procedure For Open Appendectomy

An open appendectomy is a surgical technique that removes the appendix by a single incision in the lower right abdomen. Below is a full summary of the processes required in this procedure:

1. Preparation: Before the operation, the patient is given general anesthesia to ensure that they remain asleep and pain-free during the process. The surgical team then sterilizes and drapes the operative site to provide a sterile environment.

2. Incision: The surgeon creates a single incision in the lower right abdomen, usually approximately 2 to 4 inches long. This incision permits the physician to reach the appendix and its surrounding tissues.

3. Exploration: After making the incision, the surgeon carefully examines the abdominal cavity to find the appendix. In other circumstances, if the appendix is inflamed and hidden behind other organs, the surgeon may need to gently shift these organs aside to reach it.

4. Isolation and Removal: After locating the appendix, the surgeon gently separates it from the surrounding tissue and blood arteries. The physician next uses surgical equipment to remove the appendix from the body. The base of the appendix is tied off, and the appendix is then separated from the remainder of the intestine.

5. After removing the appendix, the surgeon heals the wound with sutures or surgical staples. In rare circumstances, a drain may be inserted near the surgical site to collect excess fluid or blood.

6. Recovery: The patient is then transported to the recovery room and attentively observed while they awaken from anesthesia. Pain medication may be used to alleviate any pain after surgery.

7. Postoperative Care: After the patient is completely awake and stable, they are sent to a hospital room for continued supervision. Throughout the recuperation phase, the surgical team will offer advice on wound care, food, and activity limits.

When conducted by a skilled surgical team, an open appendectomy is a simple treatment with few complications. However, like with any operation, there are dangers such as infection, bleeding, and anesthesia-related complications. Patients should carefully follow their surgeon's instructions and report any unexpected symptoms or problems after surgery.

Step-By-Step Procedure For Laparoscopic Appendectomy

A laparoscopic appendectomy is a minimally invasive surgical technique that removes the appendix via numerous tiny incisions in the abdomen.

Below is a full summary of the processes required in this procedure:

1. Preparation: Similar to an open appendectomy, the patient is given general anesthesia to ensure they remain asleep and pain-free during the process. The surgical team then sterilizes and drapes the operative site to provide a sterile environment.

2. Trocar insertion: Rather than creating a single major incision, the surgeon creates numerous tiny incisions in the belly, each of which is less than an inch long. Trocars, which are long, thin tubes with valves, are introduced into the incisions. These trocars function as portals for the surgical tools and cameras utilized in the process.

3. Insufflation: Once the trocars are in place, carbon dioxide gas is injected into the abdominal cavity to provide room for the surgeon to operate. The surgeon can better see the internal organs when the abdomen is inflated.

4. Laparoscopic insertion: A tiny tube with a camera and light source attached is introduced via one of the trocars. The camera projects a magnified image of the abdominal organs onto a monitor in the operating room, enabling the surgeon to look inside the body without creating a big incision.

5. Exploration and Identification: Using the laparoscope, the surgeon searches the abdominal cavity for the appendix. Once the appendix has been found, the surgeon delicately moves the laparoscopic tools to isolate and remove it.

6. Isolation and Removal: The surgeon utilizes specialized laparoscopic devices, such as graspers and scissors, to gently separate the appendix from the surrounding tissue and blood arteries. The base of the appendix is then tied off, and the appendix is extracted from the body via one of the trocar incisions.

7. Closure: Once the appendix has been removed, any bleeding is stopped, and the trocar incisions are closed with sutures or surgical adhesive. Because the incisions are tiny, they usually don't need stitches and heal rapidly with little scarring.

8. Recovery and Postoperative Care: The patient is transferred to the recovery room and attentively observed when they awaken from anesthesia. Pain medication may be used to alleviate any pain after surgery. Patients may generally go home the same day or after a brief hospital stay, depending on their specific recovery.

Laparoscopic appendectomy has various benefits over open surgery, including smaller incisions, reduced post-operative discomfort, shorter hospital stays, and faster recovery periods. However, it may not be appropriate for many individuals, particularly those who have complex appendicitis or other abdominal disorders. As with any surgical operation, there are dangers such as infection, bleeding, and organ damage. Before having a laparoscopic appendectomy, patients should explore their choices with their surgeon and consider the possible advantages and dangers.

Anaesthesia And Pain Management During Surgery

Anesthesia and pain control are critical components of all surgical procedures, including appendectomy. It guarantees that the patient is comfortable and painless during the surgery. Anesthesia is a medical intervention that causes a reversible lack of feeling, enabling surgeons to conduct operations without causing pain to the patient. Appendectomy is normally performed under general anesthesia.

Before the operation, an anesthesiologist will assess the patient's medical history, current health state, and any drug allergies or sensitivities. This evaluation aids in the determination of the most suitable anesthesia regimen for the person. General anesthesia is delivered using intravenous (IV) medicines and inhalation agents.

These medicines affect the central nervous system, resulting in unconsciousness and muscular relaxation.

Once the patient is anesthetized, a breathing tube may be introduced to guarantee sufficient oxygenation during the surgery. The anesthesiologist continuously checks the patient's vital signs during the procedure to guarantee their safety and well-being. In addition to pain relief, anesthesia stops the patient from moving or feeling reflex reactions that might disrupt the surgical procedure.

In addition to anesthesia, pain management measures are used to reduce discomfort during and after surgery. This may include administering analgesic drugs before, during, and after the surgery. Non-opioid pain treatments like paracetamol and nonsteroidal anti-inflammatory drugs (NSAIDs) are often used to control post-operative pain and avoid the need for opioid prescriptions, which may have negative effects and lead to addiction.

Local anesthetics may also be used to numb the surgical site, giving extra pain relief while lowering the need for systemic drugs. Regional anesthesia procedures, such as epidural or spinal blocks, may be used in certain situations to target particular nerves and block feeling in the abdomen.

A successful appendectomy requires effective anesthesia and pain control, which ensures the patient's comfort and safety throughout the surgical procedure.

Duration And Expectations For The Procedure

The length of an appendectomy surgery varies based on many variables, including the surgical method employed, the severity of the appendicitis, and any complicating conditions present. A laparoscopic appendectomy, which is the most frequent procedure, usually takes 30 minutes to an hour to accomplish.

Open appendectomy operations might take somewhat longer, often ranging from 45 to 90 minutes.

Throughout the process, the surgical team takes a methodical approach to remove the inflamed appendix while minimizing harm to surrounding tissues. For laparoscopic appendectomy, the surgeon makes tiny incisions in the belly, while open surgery requires a bigger incision. In laparoscopic surgeries, a laparoscope—a thin, flexible tube with a camera and surgical equipment attached—is placed into one of the incisions to enable the surgeon to see the interior tissues of the abdomen.

The surgeon delicately separates the appendix from its attachments to surrounding tissues and blood vessels using specialized equipment. Once liberated, the appendix is ligated (tied off) to minimize bleeding before being removed from the abdomen. After visualizing and gaining access to the abdominal cavity, the surgeon removes the appendix via a bigger incision.

Throughout the surgery, the surgical team strictly follows aseptic measures to reduce the risk of infection. Any contaminated or irritated tissues are carefully handled and removed, and the abdominal cavity is rinsed with a sterile saline solution to eliminate any debris or germs.

Patients having appendectomy might anticipate some discomfort and soreness after the operation, which can be treated with pain medication as required. Most patients may resume regular activities within a few days to a week after surgery, however intense physical activity should be avoided during the early recovery period.

Overall, the appendectomy technique is a very simple surgical intervention with a high success rate and low complication rates when done by skilled surgeons in suitable clinical conditions. With advances in surgical procedures and anesthesia protocols, patients may undergo appendectomy with confidence, knowing that their pain and suffering will be adequately controlled and that their recovery will be quick and uncomplicated.

CHAPTER 7

Post-Operative Care

Immediate Post-Operative Care

Following an appendectomy, the patient is sent to the recovery room, where they are carefully observed by medical personnel. This period is critical because it enables healthcare workers to ensure that the patient awakens safely after anesthesia and that their vital signs stay stable. In the recovery room, nurses and physicians will constantly monitor the patient's heart rate, blood pressure, breathing rate, and oxygen saturation.

Patients may feel sleepy, confused, or even sick as the anesthesia wears off. It is usual for patients to have a dry mouth, a sore throat (due to the breathing tube used during surgery), and some pain at the surgical site. During this time, medical personnel will regularly check the patient's pain level and provide pain treatment as required. The patient's surgical dressing and incision site will also be checked for symptoms of infection or excessive bleeding.

Pain Management And Medication

Effective pain management is an essential component of postoperative treatment. Initially, pain may be treated using intravenous (IV) drugs administered in the recovery room. When the patient is stable and able to take oral drugs, the pain treatment plan usually shifts to oral pain relievers. Nonsteroidal anti-inflammatory medicines (NSAIDs) such as ibuprofen and paracetamol, as well as harsher pain relievers such as opioids, are often prescribed.

Patients should closely follow the recommended drug schedule and dosage to successfully manage pain and prevent possible consequences such as opioid addiction or overdose. It is also critical to document any adverse effects from pain drugs, such as nausea, constipation, or dizziness, and report them to your healthcare physician. Non-pharmacological pain management approaches, such as cold packs, appropriate posture, and relaxation exercises, may also help relieve discomfort.

Wound Care And Hygiene

Proper wound care and cleanliness are critical for promoting healing and preventing infections after an appendectomy. The surgical site has to be kept clean and dry. Patients are frequently instructed not to shower for the first 24-48 hours after surgery. Following this interval, gently clean the wound with moderate soap and water, being careful not to scrape the region. To avoid touching the wound, blot it dry with a clean cloth.

The dressing over the incision should be changed according to the healthcare team's recommendations, usually once a day or if it gets moist or unclean. Patients should carefully clean their hands before and after touching the wound to avoid infection. If stereo-strips (tiny sticky strips) or surgical glue were used, they should be kept in place until they come off naturally or are removed by a medical professional.

Signs Of Complications To Watch For

Monitoring for symptoms of problems is an important part of postoperative treatment. Patients and carers should be aware of any signs that may signal a problem that requires medical treatment. Common indicators of problems include:

• Check for signs of infection, such as increased redness, swelling, temperature, or discharge from the incision. Fever, chills, or increased discomfort around the surgery site may also suggest an infection.

• Report any substantial or persistent bleeding from the wound to your healthcare physician immediately.

• Wound dehiscence is when the surgical wound reopens. Signs include the wound being open or gaping, with or without drainage.

• Pain and swelling in the legs may suggest a blood clot (deep vein thrombosis). Look for swelling, redness, or soreness in your legs.

• Evaluate persistent or severe discomfort.

• Persistent nausea, vomiting, difficulty passing gas or feces, and abdominal pain may indicate ileus or bowel blockage.

Patients should be advised to seek medical attention if they exhibit any of these symptoms. Early diagnosis and treatment of complications are critical for a successful recovery.

CHAPTER 8

Recovery And Rehabilitation.

Typical Recovery Timeline

Recovering following an appendectomy is an individual journey, but there are certain typical milestones to anticipate along the road. Immediately after surgery, you will most likely spend some time in the recovery room while the anesthesia wears off. Once you are awake and stable, you will be transferred to a standard hospital room. The first day or two after surgery is usually spent managing discomfort and keeping an eye out for problems.

Within a day or two, you may begin to feel more like yourself, but you should still take it easy. Walking around the hospital room or hallway may help avoid blood clots and improve your recuperation. By the end of the first week, you may be allowed to return home, depending on your general health and the kind of surgery you had.

Once you get home, be sure to carefully follow your doctor's recommendations. You may still feel pain, particularly while moving or coughing. You will gradually recover energy and vigor. Most patients can resume modest activities within a few weeks, although it may take longer to feel fully recovered.

Activity Restrictions And Guidelines

While recovering after an appendectomy, it's critical to listen to your body and avoid overexertion. Your doctor will most likely offer specific advice depending on your unique circumstances, but here are some broad tips:

· For the first two weeks post-surgery, avoid lifting anything more than 10 pounds to minimize abdominal strain.

• Take it easy: Even if you feel better, don't push yourself too much. Stick to mild activities like walking and avoid hard activities until your doctor gives you the okay.

• Follow incision care recommendations, including monitoring for infection and adhering to doctor-recommended cleaning and dressing methods.

• Listen to your body: If you encounter pain or discomfort, call your doctor immediately.

Nutritional And Dietary Recommendations

A balanced diet is vital for promoting your body's recovery process after surgery. Here are some nutrition and food advice for your appendectomy recovery:

• Stay hydrated by drinking lots of fluids, particularly water, to avoid constipation and aid recovery.

• Focus on fiber: Consume fiber-rich meals including fruits, vegetables, whole grains, and legumes to maintain healthy digestion.

• To avoid intestinal overload, eat little, regular meals rather than big ones.

• Avoid items that induce gas and bloating, such as beans, cabbage, and carbonated drinks, since they may be unpleasant during recovery.

Follow-Up Visits And Long-Term Care

Following your appendectomy, you will need to schedule follow-up consultations with your doctor to check your recovery and ensure that you are recovering appropriately. These checkups may include physical examinations, blood testing, or imaging studies to rule out any issues.

In the long run, it is important to monitor your health and get medical assistance if you have symptoms such as chronic abdomen discomfort, fever, or vomiting.

CHAPTER 9

Complications And Risks

Common Complications Include Infection, Bleeding, And Abscess

Appendectomy, like other surgical procedures, has risks and consequences. The most frequent consequences include infection, hemorrhage, and abscess development.

Infection might develop at the site of the incision or throughout the abdominal cavity. This might be seen as redness, swelling, warmth, or discharge at the incision site. Patients with more severe conditions may feel fever, chills, and greater discomfort. Prompt detection and treatment of infection are critical for preventing its spread and reducing its effect on recovery.

Appendectomy complications could include bleeding. While some bleeding is normal during surgery, excessive bleeding during or after the treatment may lead to issues including anemia or the development of blood clots. Significant bleeding may cause dizziness, lightheadedness, or a fast heart rate. Medical staff must regularly monitor patients for indications of bleeding and respond quickly if required.

Abscess development is a possible issue that develops when pus collects in the abdominal cavity, usually due to infection. An abscess may cause chronic stomach discomfort, fever, and a palpable lump in the belly. Imaging tests, such as ultrasonography or CT scans, may be required to confirm the diagnosis. Drainage of the abscess may be necessary to avoid future problems.

Rare Yet Serious Complications

While uncommon, appendectomy may cause significant consequences that need emergency medical treatment. This may include:

• Peritonitis is a serious illness that affects the lining of the abdominal cavity (peritoneum). It may happen if the appendix ruptures during surgery or if appendicitis is not treated promptly enough. Peritonitis symptoms may include severe stomach discomfort, fever, nausea, and vomiting.

• Surgery may cause accidental injury to neighboring organs such as the intestines, bladder, and blood arteries. This may lead to severe difficulties and may need further surgical treatments to fix.

• Scar tissue formation following surgery might cause intestinal obstruction. This might result in symptoms including stomach discomfort, bloating, constipation, and vomiting.

While these consequences are uncommon, people should be aware of the risks and seek medical assistance if they develop any worrying symptoms after an appendectomy.

How To Identify And Respond To Complications

Early detection of problems is critical for prompt treatment and best results. Patients should be aware of any indications or symptoms that might signal a problem, such as:

• Chronic or increasing stomach discomfort.

• Fever.

• Chills.

• Redness, swelling, or drainage around the incision site.

• Nausea or vomiting.

• Changes in bowel habits.

• Difficulty urinating.

If any of these symptoms appear, patients should contact their healthcare physician right once for additional examination and advice. Depending on the severity of the issue, other tests or procedures may be required to decide the best course of treatment.

Preventive Measures And Risk Management

While it is difficult to remove all hazards connected with appendectomy, there are various preventative treatments and risk reduction methods that may help reduce the possibility of problems.

• Before surgery, patients should have a comprehensive medical assessment to check their general health and identify any risk factors that may lead to difficulties.

• Antibiotic treatment before surgery may lower the incidence of postoperative infections.

• Laparoscopic appendectomy, which uses tiny incisions, a camera, and specialized equipment to remove the appendix, is less intrusive and reduces the risk of problems like infection and bleeding compared to standard open surgery.

• Close monitoring: After surgery, patients should be regularly observed for any symptoms of problems and receive appropriate treatments as required.

Healthcare practitioners may assist protect the safety and well-being of patients having appendectomy by using these preventative measures and responding quickly to any issues that develop.

CHAPTER 10

Appendectomy In Special Populations

Appendectomy In Children

Appendectomy, or surgical removal of the appendix, is a frequent operation for children. The appendix is a tiny, tube-like organ that connects to the big intestine. Appendicitis, or inflammation of the appendix, is a somewhat frequent illness in children that needs surgical intervention.

One of the most difficult aspects of doing an appendectomy on a kid is correctly identifying appendicitis. Children may not always display typical appendicitis symptoms, such as stomach pain in the lower right quadrant. Instead, patients may feel nonspecific stomach pain, lack of appetite, or nausea, making diagnosis more difficult. Furthermore, young toddlers may struggle to appropriately explain their symptoms.

When appendicitis is suspected in a kid, quick medical attention is required to avoid complications such as appendiceal rupture. Physical examination, blood testing, and imaging procedures such as an ultrasound or CT scan may all be part of the diagnosis process. Once appendicitis is diagnosed, surgical removal of the appendix is usually advised.

Appendectomy in children is often done using less invasive procedures, such as laparoscopic surgery. This method includes creating tiny abdominal incisions through which specialized surgical equipment and a camera are introduced. The surgeon then visualizes the appendix on a monitor before removing it with little devices.

Minimally invasive appendectomy has various benefits for children, including shorter hospital stays, quicker recovery periods, and a lower risk of problems such as wound infection. However, not all children may be eligible for laparoscopic surgery, depending on the severity of the appendicitis and the existence of underlying medical issues.

In conclusion, appendectomy in minors requires careful evaluation of diagnostic issues, surgical strategy, and postoperative care. Early detection of appendicitis symptoms and timely medical assessment are critical to achieving optimal outcomes in children having appendectomy.

Appendectomy While Pregnant

Appendectomy during pregnancy is a surgical technique used to remove an inflamed appendix in pregnant women who have been diagnosed with appendicitis. Appendicitis is a disorder that causes inflammation of the appendix, which is a tiny pouch situated at the intersection of the small and large intestines.

Performing an appendectomy during pregnancy involves special problems because of worries about the mother's and fetus's safety. Appendicitis is one of the most frequent non-obstetric surgical emergencies during pregnancy, necessitating immediate diagnosis and treatment to avoid consequences including appendiceal rupture and peritonitis.

Appendicitis during pregnancy may be difficult to diagnose since symptoms overlap with common pregnant discomforts such as nausea, vomiting, and abdominal pain. To prevent problems, diagnosis and treatment should not be delayed.

When a pregnant woman is suspected of having appendicitis, she may have a full assessment that includes a physical examination, blood tests, and imaging procedures like as ultrasound or MRI to confirm the diagnosis. Once appendicitis is diagnosed, surgical removal of the inflamed appendix is usually indicated to avoid rupture and peritonitis.

Appendectomy during pregnancy may be done open or laparoscopically, depending on the severity of the appendix, gestational age, and maternal status. Laparoscopic appendectomy, which includes making tiny incisions in the belly and using specialized equipment, is often chosen when possible because of its least invasive nature and speedier recovery periods.

However, the choice to conduct an appendectomy during pregnancy must include both the risks and advantages to the mother and the fetus. The surgical team will make efforts to reduce possible hazards, such as monitoring the fetal heart rate throughout surgery and administering adequate anesthesia to guarantee maternal and fetal safety.

Appendectomy during pregnancy necessitates careful evaluation of the specific difficulties and hazards involved. Early diagnosis, adequate surgical technique, and thorough monitoring of both the mother and the fetus are critical for favorable results in pregnant women having appendectomy.

Appendectomy In Elderly Patients

Appendectomy in elderly individuals requires special considerations owing to age-related physiological changes and the presence of comorbidities that might impair surgical results. Appendicitis, or inflammation of the appendix, may occur in the elderly, although it may manifest differently than in younger people.

Elderly persons with appendicitis may feel stomach pain, nausea, vomiting, and fever, although these symptoms may be less severe or appear differently than in younger people. Furthermore, senior people may have additional medical disorders, such as diabetes, hypertension, or heart disease, complicating the diagnosis and treatment of appendicitis.

When appendicitis is suspected in an older adult, quick medical attention is required to avoid complications such as perforation and peritonitis. Physical examinations, blood tests, and imaging procedures such as CT scans or ultrasounds may be used to confirm the diagnosis.

The surgical care of appendicitis in older adults may include an open or laparoscopic appendectomy, depending on the severity of the appendix, the patient's general health state, and surgical risk. Laparoscopic appendectomy is often favored when possible owing to its less invasive nature and speedier recovery durations.

However, the choice to undertake an appendectomy on an aged patient must weigh the possible risks and advantages of surgery, taking into consideration the patient's general health state, the existence of comorbidities, and surgical risk. The surgical team will make efforts to reduce perioperative risks and provide the best possible results for elderly patients having appendectomy.

In conclusion, appendectomy in the elderly involves careful consideration of age-related changes in physiology, the existence of comorbidities, and surgical risk. Early diagnosis, effective surgical therapy, and perioperative care are critical for excellent results in older people with appendicitis.

Considerations For Patients With Other Medical Conditions

Patients with various medical issues may need particular care while having an appendectomy. Appendicitis, or inflammation of the appendix, may develop in people who have pre-existing medical disorders such as diabetes, obesity, or immunocompromised states, which might affect the diagnosis and treatment of the illness.

When appendicitis is suspected in a patient with other medical issues, further assessment, and diagnostic testing may be required to confirm the diagnosis and determine the severity of appendicitis. Blood tests, imaging examinations such as a CT scan or ultrasound, and contact with experts may be necessary to optimize care.

Surgical care of appendicitis in individuals with other medical issues may include open or laparoscopic appendectomy, depending on the severity of the appendix, the patient's general health state, and surgical risk. The surgical team will make efforts to reduce perioperative risks and provide the best possible results for these patients.

Furthermore, individuals with various medical issues may need specialized perioperative care to meet their unique requirements and reduce possible consequences. This may involve optimizing medical conditions before to surgery, administering appropriate antibiotics, and monitoring patients after surgery to ensure a quick recovery.

Prompt diagnosis, interdisciplinary treatment, and individualized perioperative care are critical for excellent results in these patients.

Conclusion

Knowing appendectomy is critical for both medical professionals and the general population. This thorough reference has offered information on the anatomy, symptoms, diagnosis, and treatment of appendicitis, emphasizing the need for early detection and surgical intervention.

Appendectomy is the gold standard therapy for acute appendicitis, with a high success rate and minimal complication rates when done on time. Laparoscopic appendectomy has revolutionized surgical practices, with shorter recovery periods and fewer postoperative problems than open surgery.

However, the choice to operate should always be based on a thorough clinical review that includes the patient's history, physical examination results, and imaging investigations. Differential diagnosis should also be considered since similar diseases might lead to misdiagnosis and delayed treatment.

Furthermore, post-operative care is critical to achieving the best possible results, with a focus on pain management, early ambulation, and monitoring for potential complications such as wound infection, intra-abdominal abscess, or ileus.

Advances in medical technology and surgical procedures continue to enhance appendicitis therapy, with improved results and patient satisfaction. Nonetheless, continuous research is required to improve diagnostic algorithms, optimize treatment techniques, and investigate novel ways to manage this prevalent surgical emergency.

By understanding the complexities of appendicitis and appendectomy, healthcare practitioners may offer prompt and effective treatment, while patients can make educated choices regarding their health and well-being. Together, this information enables us to face the problems of appendicitis with confidence and competence.

THE END

www.ingramcontent.com/pod-product-compliance
Lightning Source LLC
Chambersburg PA
CBHW051908250726
48659CB00002B/545